USING NATURAL OILS TO REFRESH, RESTORE
AND REJUVENATE YOUR SKIN

SIMPLY OILS

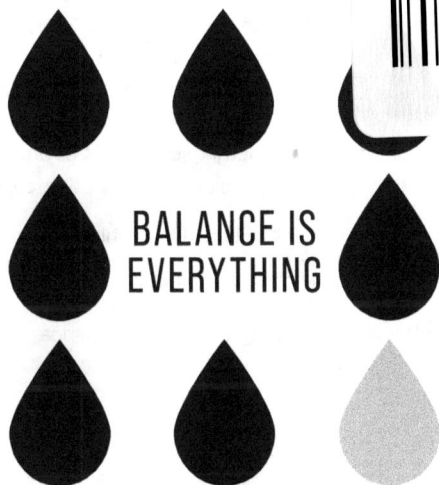

BALANCE IS
EVERYTHING

I0123250

DR. KALLY PAPANTONIOU

Simply Oils

Copyright © 2022

Published by Elevate Publishing

ISBN 979-8-9862830-9-8

Printed in the United States of America

I dedicate this book to my supportive husband and two loving boys. Thank you for making this life so amazing, and always standing by my side.

CONTENTS

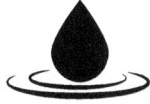

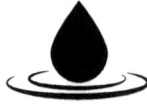

Simply Oils

An insider's review on the use of oils in skincare by New York Dermatologist and oil enthusiast Dr. Kally Papantoniou. Many do not know that oils have been used for millennia in skin care, and only fell out of favor when it became a fad perpetuated by big industry that skin care products are best if they are oil-free. How did we move away from oils in skin care? When did this become a bad thing? Oils are not the only public enemy in social history ("fat free" diet crazes, "sweet n low/artificial sweeteners" instead of sugar or honey). Remember when women were told to use baby formula and canned milk over breast milk, etc. We often move away from nature in place of industrialized monetized replacements. Back to our roots. The movement of peoples to make social decisions to go back to basics, closer to nature, and appreciate how mankind has been living for beyond centuries. Here we recognize the importance of oils in skincare and how we can help improve skin conditions and slow the aging process.

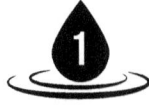

"An Introduction"

This is not an encyclopedic book about oils. If you are looking for a book detailing oils with scientific resources, keep looking, there are plenty out there. This is a book about the passion of one dermatologist to provide the best skin care for health and anti-aging, and that just happens to have a lot to do with the use of natural oils. If that is something in which you might be interested, then you are in the right place. You can be sure that as technology improves, many of the treatments that we currently offer for skin rejuvenation will have improved as well, but what I can say for certain is that the common sense, bare-bone approach that I have for skin care will still hold true and be irreplaceable.

Who am I to tell you anything about skincare? Well, I get my qualifications from my medical degree as a dermatologist; but it goes beyond that. My fascination with all things skin began for me when I was just a little girl. I was one of these kids who just knew they wanted to be a doctor when they grow up, I just didn't know what kind or what it really meant. But while other kids my age were making pizzas out of play-doh, I was making a play model of a layer of skin covering bones and blood vessels on my mother's leg while she watched TV . . . and then I performed surgery on this "skin" with her metal nail filer and cuticle cutters . . . years later this memory would become the opening to my essay for my medical school application. It started off kind of like this: "The young doctor made the initial incision of the skin with the scalpel. The skin cancer was successfully removed. The skin was repaired by closing with an extra layer of play-doh, and the nail filer was put back on the surgical tray." It was a playful memory for me and I suppose the reader figured any kid weird enough to do that might make an "OK" doctor one day. Ha.

I also happen to come from a family that has dealt with many different skin conditions, such as psoriasis, eczema, and acne, oh my. Meanwhile, when I was a child, I had no idea what exactly any of it was that I was seeing. I grew up wondering what on earth my grandfather was scratching and pretty much carving away at with a knife on the backs of his gnarled scaling hands. I had no idea this was psoriasis, and, to be honest, I bet none of the adults around me knew either. He was an immigrant from Greece, escaping from the border of Northern Greece that was controlled by Communist Albania, bringing his wife and 5 children to the United States in a manner very similar to many other political refugees. They immigrated with no money or support, but they had their family and work ethic with survival being the only option for all of them.

My grandfather was tough as nails, and such a naturally intelligent person who only got to attend school up to the 4th grade. Yet, he learned how to read and write English, and had a strong interest in history and his family. He once said if he could do it all over again, he would have been a professor. My grandfather did love talking so much and he was a very patient man, he would have made a great professor. This guy would flip through the White Pages back in the 1990s, and he would cold call people with Greek names just to have a conversation with them, I mean, who does that? Yet, when my mother told him she wanted to be a nurse in the late 60s he said "No, you will be a mother." Times were different, you could say. Women were expected to be mothers and stay at home in our family.

And my late Aunt Ginny, from the same side of the family, was a firecracker of a human being. She was full of life, merriment, bursts of anger, and she was one of the absolute funniest, most beautiful people you ever are lucky enough to meet, let alone be related to. The first pimples I remember extracting were my Aunt Ginny's, she was a smoker and always had crazy large clogged pores around her ears. She was a hair dresser/chain smoker, and I was always fascinated by her fake nails and blonde hair that was always perfectly hair-sprayed. She was so happy to have me take out her clogged pores, and from a young age I learned what a little creepy dermatologist I was–and this predated the "Pimple Popper" show by about 30 years. But these were ginormous deep acne pockets, not for the weak of heart or stomach, LOL. My aunt also suffered from scaling in her ears, that she would scratch and pick at them with a toothpick, and this would in turn leave her with scar tissue in her ear canal. I now know that what she had was a form of eczema that was left untreated. Later in life, my aunt would come to me for the treatment of a melanoma that I diagnosed and excised for her. My child play came to full circle with my aunt actually needing me to be her dermatologist.

As an early teenager, I had moderate acne, which unfortunately for me started a bit earlier than with my peers. This absolutely was not cool. I was walking around with a forehead covered in little bumps and blackheads, crusty scabs in all different stages of healing because I was also a picker. Not to mention, my mother who was a bit of a bohemian and one to underplay almost everything . . . for example, my sister once hurt her arm when we were around 10 years old, and she said, "Mom, it hurts a lot when I lift my arm." You would think that she would examine it a bit herself, maybe even suggest that we should see a doctor. My mother's actual reply was, "Ok, so don't lift your arm." Now, if my sister was 10 years-old, I must have only been about 7, and at that age I even sensed that there was something off with this situation. LOL. So, basically, she was not an alarmist, to say the least. My mom would pop my pimples, and my sisters and I would often pick each other's pimples similar to a group of chimpanzees picking at each other on a nature documentary; we were officially a family of pickers. I have no idea how I don't have any scars from that time, but I am super fortunate that I did not have cystic acne, otherwise I would have most likely been left with battle wounds from these years. And as you can imagine, my dermatology appointments for acne were virtually non-existent. I was totally bullied by my peers for my acne, who were not at all understanding. This experience has turned me into a very empathetic practitioner, as I can try to understand how some of my patients feel about their skin and how this impacts daily life.

It is all about feelings in dermatology. Everything that can basically go wrong in dermatology can affect your feelings. It is unique in that unlike the other fields of medicine, in which most of the conditions being treated do not leave the patient with something that has to be shown on your skin for the world to see. When I finally did go to medical school, and had my first lecture in dermatology, it was like Pandora's box opening, or a puzzle piece showing up that I had been searching for, without my realizing. I finally had found my purpose, my fit in medicine.

I did most of my training in Brooklyn and on Long Island, with rotations that involved diverse training hospitals and private clinics that truly offered such a wide spectrum of patient populations, and the skin conditions that arise within them. I stand on the shoulders of true dermatology giants. My chairman was the late Dr. Alan Shalita, who gave me the chance to become a dermatologist. He was a brilliant, warm man who dedicated his life to establishing our dermatology department at SUNY Downstate. He once joked that he was finally able to say my last name, which was my maiden name at the time, Tzezailidis, and when he announced my name at our match ceremony, he said he now had to practice and "relearn my new last name Papantoniou, which is just as difficult to say. He was a great man, and I learned so much from him. Dr. Shalita was known for his groundbreaking research and approach to treating acne, his work with isotretinoin has helped pave the way for the treatment of cystic acne, and I am proud to have been a resident at SUNY Downstate.

The other mentors to whom I owe so much to include my attendings, who were so gracious with their time as I shadowed their busy practices, they are some of the smartest people I have ever met. My brilliant pediatric dermatology attending and preceptor, and the dermatopathologists who taught me everything I know about pathology and the art of reading slides. They really should know that they are appreciated and have helped so many people in this life by training the future dermatologists as well as they do. Thank you.

Funny story, I wanted to show the department of dermatology how much my training meant to me, that I was graduating, and I wanted to present them with a gift that came from the heart, so I worked on creating a painting on a large canvas. I asked our lead dermatopathologist what his favorite pathology slide was to look at under the microscope, and he said his favorite slide is "molluscum." To picture what this looks like under the microscope, imagine a pomegranate cut in cross section with bright violets, reds, indigos, and pinks; this is the beauty of what molluscum looks like . . . now the actual skin condition is pretty nasty, it is, after all, a contagious virus that affects both children and adults, and can actually be sexually transmitted . . . but who am I to judge? This was his favorite slide. So, I painted it. And it was beautiful. It was time consuming. And I managed to do this while studying for the boards, and I had a 2-year-old at the time . . . just saying. Anyway, so I present him and the department with this painting that I have made. And what was his comment? "It is upside down." That is pretty much all I got. It was a bit deflating, but overall, a funny laugh to myself. I didn't do it for praise, or for thanks, I did it because deep down I know that I am incredibly lucky to have the training that I have, I am so privileged to take care of skin the way I do, to have this passed-down knowledge. So, I say thank you, again.

2

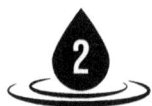

"How the Skincare Economy Left Skin Broke"

When you learn to love your skin and you start to think about it as something that needs to be taken care of, when you think of all the good things that your skin is already doing for you on a daily basis without you lifting a finger, you start to realize just how amazing your skin is and this deeper understanding may help guide you and motivate you to take care of your skin better, as you would anything that you truly cared about and loved. This means doing the right thing on a daily basis. This means taking care of your skin by cleansing it, putting the right products on it, and generally doing the best in your power to ensure that your skin is as healthy as possible. And when you do that, and your goal is to ensure that your skin is as healthy as possible, then naturally you become a magnet for finding things to do for your skin that will help it also look more youthful. The products and the methods that we apply toward maintaining healthy skin and a healthy skin barrier are the very same techniques and tips that we recommend for rejuvenating skin.

With a thorough understanding for how the skin functions, and what its needs are, we have applied our knowledge, experience, and research toward establishing the best skin care routine that will benefit most people who struggle with dry skin, sensitive skin, rosacea, and would like to help their skin stay healthy and look youthful. What is youthful skin? Youthful skin has a high abundance of healthy collagen fibers that are organized in a basket weave formation, which ensures durability and firmness to our skin. Skin that is youthful also has a balance of essential fatty acids and waxy lipids present on the outer layers; these layers help to maintain moisture within the skin and help to protect skin from outside environmental factors, and are essential for healthy skin. Youthful skin has high levels of moisture that also helps it look firm and smooth, as well. As we age, hydration levels diminish, contributing to the appearance of laxity.

Since the 1980s, there has been a change in the trend for skin care that has let us down a path toward using oil-free products. The idea that oil-free products are better for your skin has become a mainstream concept, and standard, but we will soon see how this is misguided advice that has been perpetuated by an entire industry. There are many reasons for why this has happened, and we can see similar problems such as this that have happened in other industries, where the consumer is targeted to purchase a product that is not in their best interest.

Oils really have been used in skin care traditions as far back as history has been recorded. We have evidence of the use of oils in ancient Egypt. The ancient Egyptians used oils in skin care routines and rituals. They often used oils, such as olive oil, to cleanse and moisturize their skin. The ancient Greeks also used olive oil to cleanse and moisturize their skin. One of the first recorded creams came from ancient Greece: a scientist had used beeswax in combination with olive oil to formulate a primitive cold cream. This concoction of beeswax and oil was one of the first recorded findings of a cream to be used for moisturizing. This concept was continued through centuries, where this rough prototype was refined and was implemented in many people's skin-care routine and was very helpful in maintaining a healthy barrier. It was a breakthrough idea to combine an oil with a wax-like substance to formulate a creamy product that would be easy to spread and great for skin. Today we still use waxes to make creams, but they are usually synthetic.

So why then, you might ask yourself, after thousands of years of the use of oils for skin care would we now have to say that oils are bad for your skin and you should only be using oil-free products. The explanation for why this has occurred is most likely for several reasons, but one of the most convincing is that the skin-care industry is constantly reinventing itself, and, with this, the expansion and promotion of new and improved approaches and ingredients are developed. In skin care, new and improved products will be advertised with the help of buzzwords that will help sell a product, and this is often done by inciting an emotion such as fear. In advertising, fear sells, fear of missing out, fear of doing the wrong thing, fear of not fitting in . . . and these emotions can be called upon to persuade a customer to make a purchase.

When the label says "oil-free" on a product, this

sends a message to the consumer that oil must be bad; and if they want better skin, healthier skin, they should buy this oil-free product. When a consumer reads a label, they will pick up a phrase such as "organic," "rejuvenating," "all-natural," and this can help sell a product, this can create a trend with products that will make one product more desirable than another, and can change the direction of an industry. When the "oil-free" direction started to take place and was successful, it expanded over to more products and more skin-care companies fell into line with making oil-free products. This certainly may be important in certain circumstances for people who are sensitive to oils, but not an across-the-board recommendation for the general population. And it has put a stigma on the use of oils in skin care.

Revolutionary ideas that have turned upside down what humankind has been doing for thousands of years are not unique to the skin-care industry. For example, the whole "fat free" diet craze was a concept of a fat-free food being better for a diet has been disapproved by the nutritionists and is not backed by any science. These products that are fat-free often contain synthetic compounds and high amounts of sugar in order to compensate for the loss of flavor and satisfaction that comes from having fat in the food product. Our bodies actually need fat and there are healthful fats that help our bodies function optimally, to help control cholesterol, help brain function, the list really goes on and on. But once a product has been labeled as fat free, it sent a message to the consumer that fat must be bad and this food is superior because it doesn't have fat, again instilling fear in the consumer that if they eat something else that has fat that is in it then they will become overweight. What is interesting is that people for thousands upon thousands of years have been surviving just fine and maintaining a healthy weight with healthful foods that contain fats, and now all the sudden it is bad!

How easily manipulated are we as consumers! It truly is surprising in how short of a period of time we see complete reversals of what we know to be good for our health. We know fats are good for our bodies, we know that when they eliminate the good fats from foods that they then have to replace it with sugar or artificial sweeteners in order to compensate for the taste. We know that this food, even though it's fat free, actually can increase the glycemic index and may lead, in turn, the body to create more fat storage than had the food consumed been a normal balanced treat. We also see this with sugar-free foods, with sugar being replaced by artificial sweeteners.

The "sugar-free" on the packaging makes the consumer think this is a better solution for them. After all, it is "sugar free." Sugar-free foods will often be laden with chemicals that can have other health concerns, and have not been shown to help with weight loss anyway.

This is why it is so important to consider what your skin is, to consider how it functions, how it does all the amazing things that it does for you every day and what we should be doing to help take care of it. Oil-free products, for instance, do not help maintain a healthy skin care barrier. Oil-free products will not help retain moisture in your skin. And most of these oil-free products contain synthetic compounds that are oil-like. Synthetic compounds, and oils that are artificial, do not contain the benefits of natural oils, such as antioxidants, polyphenols, and an array of short- and long-chain fatty acids that helps support healthy skin. If oils are not only safe, but essential for us to consume on a daily basis, it isn't that hard to understand just how important oils are for your skin. Remember, our skin is the largest organ of our body; it is alive, it thrives on all the nutrients that you eat; all the vitamins; all the nutrition; all the fats; all the oils, all the collagen, and all the proteins—the list goes on and on. What is amazing is that your skin is the only organ that you can directly treat with vitamins and oils and other beneficial nutrients. And it's the only organ that you can directly observe the benefits of treating. It would be silly to not treat it directly and just expect the oils that you eat and the vitamins that you take to be delivered to your skin; not that these aren't important, but why not do it directly when you have access to it every day!

After years of training and practicing as a dermatologist, I have come to understand how to best treat skin mostly from observation, trial and error, and seeing what works for patients and seeing what hasn't worked. I, too, have been influenced for many years by the industries that have dictated what the "right" way to treat skin is. I have used so-called gentle cleansers, moisturizing cleansers, and cleansers that are great for eczema, only to find that these cleansers are still, at the end of the day, gentle soaps that still wash off our natural oils and disrupt the delicate balance of our skin. If I didn't see the number of patients that I do, if I didn't treat skin conditions such as eczema and psoriasis, people with recalcitrant dry skin who do not respond to the best moisturizers and so-called gentle skin care available, I would not have come to realize the important impact cleansers have on skin conditions. Without the right cleanser, or should I say with the wrong cleanser, it doesn't matter what kind of moisturizer you use; you're never going to fully replace what your skin was making to begin with. There is no moisturizer available that will ever fully replace what your skin is meant to do, and once you have removed those oils by cleansing with the soap and you have removed the top layers of your skin by scrubbing or with exfoliating; this disrupts that barrier and there is not a moisturizer that is going to fix this. We will discuss further what the ideal skin care regimen is for maintaining a balanced moisture level and how to attain the healthiest skin possible.

It's not your fault, no one is putting the blame on you for over-washing your skin and not taking care of it the right way. We are all products of what we've been taught and we haven't watched this evolve over time, we've been born into it because this generation hasn't seen this switch in skin care guidance. We haven't seen this shift in not using oils in skin care in an obvious manner, because rather than being abrupt, it has been slow and gradual.

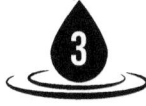

"Barriers to Skin Care"

The advice I'm going to give you may sound counterintuitive or crazy and maybe even dirty, but it's really deeply rooted in some basic common sense. My ideology in skin care is really born out of seeing what works best for patients, with an added dose of common sense for lack of better words. Modern skin care is heavily influenced by commercial products, product placement, and the ads to which we are exposed and with which we've been indoctrinated since our childhoods. Essentially the issue is that we are to clean. To squeaky clean! The way I think of it, mankind has been around a very long time, and we didn't have any running hot water or commercial soaps, it just wasn't a thing. Now, I'm not saying that we should be caveman and not bathe, but let's pull it back a little here and think about this a little bit better. And I believe that before we get into how you should wash, we should really think about how skin functions. If you really know how your skin works, then you'll fully understand why washing as though you have trudged through a toxic swamp every day may, surprisingly, not be the best thing for your skin.

Without exaggeration, I can say that when a patient is suffering with either eczema or chronic dry skin, in particular, 50% of the cases of these conditions are secondary to chronic over washing. It is not anyone's fault, and it's not your fault for doing this if you do. Part of the issue is with these widespread product placement ads for shampoos and body washes that feature women scrubbing in the shower and sudsing up. So, by really lathering up with soap from head to toe, you know that "you're not fully clean until you're Zest fully clean." We've all seen these commercials and can sing to the tunes, and we've seen the commercials for Dial antibacterial soap . . . But the other core rationale for these common behaviors is that for so many it is just tradition. Those who are descendants of people who come from many parts of the world that may have even been hotter and more humid may be more inclined to have such customs. In countries where it's hotter more and humid, people just tend to wash more frequently. In fact, I'll often meet a patient who is either from this type of climate or their family comes from there, those who come from more of a tropical climate will often continue skin care practices as though they still live there even though they live in New York where it's not a particularly humid climate, especially not in the winter months. Funny thing is a lot of these people will still be bathing twice a day, maybe even 3 times a day, and good luck to me for trying to explain to this person that they shouldn't be bathing so often.

When you've been brought up a certain way, it's an anathema to not clean this way. To add insult to injury, people also use washcloths, sponges, loofahs, and scrubbing brushes, which truly work against everything your skin is trying to do for you. My theory for how washcloths even came into the bathroom and the shower stall is that many years ago, without running water, maybe once a week or maybe twice, when people needed to bathe, they would have a basin of water and they would use a washcloth dip it into the water and apply some homemade soap then they would use that washcloth all over their body because that's what they had; they didn't have a bathtub, they didn't have running water, maybe they didn't live by running stream. But this washcloth mentality has been passed down for generations, and when you have easy access to warm running water and you have soap, you really don't need to wash with a cloth like that all over your body, especially if you have a skin issue. I do wish to point out that this advice isn't necessarily universal, because there are certain people who do have skin that is way more tolerant and they might do fine and their skin might perform great with twice-daily washing and scrubbing with a washcloth or a loofah. But I'm going to say that most people probably cannot wash like that without having dry skin, and without finding the need to constantly moisturize with commercial moisturizers.

So why is washing with soap and a washcloth and scrubbing and sudsing a problem? In order to really understand the problem. you really have to think about how the skin functions and what it needs to sustain its processes. Now, your skin is really smart, it's truly brilliant, it does 1 million things every day for you that you don't even know about. Some of the basic functions and essential structures within your skin help to maintain an amazing barrier that protects you from the outside world. Your skin is structured similarly to a brick-and-mortar wall, the skin cells are held together by waxy lipids and delicate connections between the cells that help keep your skin together and create a shield protecting the deeper layers. The waxy lipids help retain moisture in your skin and help keep the skin smooth, which prevents cracking and flaking. Tiny cracks and fissures in the skin can be a kink in your armor, allowing viruses, bacteria, and fungus to enter and grow, leading to many different infections. With a virus, you can develop warts or herpes, which can be chronic or recurrent. If bacteria enter the skin, a dangerous bacterial infection known as cellulitis may occur and requires antibiotics and sometimes even hospitalization. A fungal infection can occur when a fungal spore enters. This is called candida intertrigo or tinea corporis, aka ring worm. In people who have dryer skin or suffer from conditions such as psoriasis or eczema, which causes a defect in the skin barrier, we will see increased infections such as the ones I've mentioned. It is not uncommon that they can get in the way of treating those conditions.

The outer-most layers of skin are compacted dead skin cells and waxy lipids; the deeper layers are made of live cells. The living cells are also connected together with a delicate network of fibers that hold structure and provide pathways for cells to communicate. Underneath this cellular layer is then a zone where all the collagen fibers and connective tissues are located. This is the part that makes our skin the strongest and helps to hold it together and hold down those more delicate upper layers of skin cells. This is called the dermal layer and it is also the layer of skin that contains most of your skin's nerve endings and blood vessels. Below the dermal layer is where you'll find fat.

So, in the most basic terms, these are the 3 layers of your skin and this is how they function. So, I ask again, what are you accomplishing when you wash with a washcloth? When we wash with a washcloth, especially a white cloth, you might look at it and say "oh gross, look at how dirty I am, look at all that brown stuff on there, that's disgusting, so much dirt just came off my body!" Yeah, that would be wrong. Those are just skin cells that have been scrubbed off that look that color because whether you are very dark skinned or you have a more medium skin tone, when you when you scrub your skin, of course the skin has some pigment to it, it has some natural color to it, so it may definitely look like you just scrubbed off a ton of dirt but all you really did was scrub off the top layers of your skin. And, can I remind you that your skin worked really hard to make that protective layer? As you get older, it doesn't make skin cells so great anymore, that process really slows. So, you've succeeded in removing dead top layers, and to top it off, the soap that most likely was on that washcloth also succeeded in washing away your natural oils. So now what are we left with? We're left with skin that's all dried out and has a kink in the armor because you removed that top layer that was your armor; you know, the one that was protecting you from the outside environment. You end up with microscopic breaks in the skin and a thinner top layer, so your skin dries out like a desert and is more vulnerable to all the different things you might find in your environment.

What I didn't mention is when you have chronic breaks in the skin surface and then an impacted barrier such as this, that you can also acquire allergies to the environment more easily. Allergies may be acquired more readily because what was normally restricted to the outside world on the surface of your skin now gets introduced to the deeper layers in your skin so you're going to have an increase in allergies to skin care products, ingredients, perfumes, detergent, dander . . . the list really goes on and on. No matter what moisturizer you put on, it will never fully replace what your skin was making, it just doesn't work like that.

There is no moisturizer that will fully replicate what your skin was making, nor will it be deeply integrated within your skin the way that it should be, the way that your skin already makes it. That is why, more often than not, when I am treating a patient and they tell me that their skin is super dry and it doesn't get better even though they are using all the best moisturizers, it just can't get any better . . . My first questions are not about what moisturizer is being used, it's with what are you washing? How are you washing? Do use a washcloth? How many times a day are you washing like that? Because that's the logical train of thought for the line of questioning, because I know that even if I give them the moisturizer that I think works the best, if I don't treat the underlying problem, this person is never going to get better. And that's a really hard thing to drive home to somebody. Most of these people look at me like I'm crazy, and dirty, and don't know what I'm talking about. It actually ends up being a pretty funny conversation, to be honest, and I fully enjoy it. But I think you can tell I'm super passionate about it, knowledgeable, and experienced, so I can comfortably recommend a change in the skin care routine that I know will benefit the patient. Sadly, I also know that no one else is probably going to sit there and take the time to explain this and help guide them and show them the right way to take care of their skin. And it's especially important when I have a patient who is taking care of a newborn baby or a young child, that has different skin than the mother or the father, maybe the parents are totally fine and never had any issues with dry skin or eczema, but the kid has skin care issues. So, it's hard to explain to the caregivers, but it is so Important and it's the most helpful advice that I can give because once I do that, their skin will always be better for it and perhaps they will still need a little prescription cream here and there to help control a flareup, but I can guarantee that it will be less frequent and it'll be less severe when there is a flareup of an underlying skin condition.

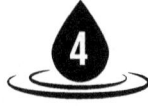

"A Drop of Love"

n an age where so much is known about molecular genetics, the ins and outs of how skin functions, how skin disease occurs, and how skin conditions can be easily modified and improved with skincare practices, I am astounded every day when I have to have "the discussion" with my patients, about how they should be taking care of their skin. I am often met with some level of confrontation, disbelief, or straight up bewilderment when I try to explain the best ways to take care of one's skin and that of their family's skin. I am a practicing Cosmetic and Medical Dermatologist, and I find myself sounding sometimes too similar to a broken record most days, giving the same advice to my patients who have been unknowingly led astray by media, marketing, and cosmetic companies, and very often their own mother's on how to take care of their skin. In this book, I hope to spread the word to help undo some of this misinformation, and to hopefully bring some relief to those of you who are struggling to feel better, and have healthier skin. The answers are truly not so complex, as they are common sense, but nonetheless I find that all the patients who have crossed my path, and were struggling, have returned with gratitude and are more in control of their skin than ever before. So read on, if you have an open mind, a sense of humor, and are wondering why your skin is no better, even after seeing one or even two Dermatologists.

Are you Squeaky Clean? I am starting off with probably one of the most difficult subjects to broach upon with my patients. But I will give actual examples of how the conversation goes with the patient, and hopefully this will give you a little background information on why I take the time out of my busy schedule to really ingrain these ideas into the patient during their visit. I find that it is my duty as their dermatologist, to educate you, the patient on how to be in charge of your own skin. It is the case that often patients will come in for a consultation, and will already have had a diagnosis of eczema for years, and when I discuss their skin care routines, I am so surprised to find that apparently, they were never informed on how to take care of their skin properly, or perhaps they weren't listening . . . When I am evaluating a new patient that has a history of eczema, dry skin, psoriasis, or possibly another skin condition I first discuss at length the everyday basics, and try to be a bit of a detective with unveiling what skin practices they have already set. If instead I offered only advice, and told the patient what to do, without involving them, or first finding out what it is they are doing, the rate of compliance is much lower.

For example, this is usually how the questioning will go, and I will ask them, wait for the answer, run through all my questions before I comment. You can run through the questions yourself, and think of your answers to them (try to be honest with yourself).

1. How many times per day do you bathe?
2. Do you lather up really well with soap?
3. Are you using a wash cloth or a sponge?
4. What type of cleanser are you using?
5. When you are done, do you moisturize?
6. Do you finish your skincare with a body oil?

Now let's look at how my follow-up response is to the answers of those same questions.

1. How many times per day do you bathe?

I ask how many times per day, this way if they are bathing 2 or three times per day, I have a higher chance of hearing the truth, as opposed to just didactically telling the patient to shower no more than once daily. Often the number of times can be cultural as well, depending on what part of the world the patient is from, bathing 2 or three times a day may be customary. I will ask that they try to cut down their bathing to once daily, explaining that over washing makes it very difficult for your skin to keep up, and it will be very difficult to prevent it from drying out with these habits.

And on the opposite spectrum, there are people who have been instructed to only bathe every other day or a few times per week, because they have a history of eczema. I spend a minute here, if they do tell me they don't bathe every day because they were told it was bad to do, I explain: "The water is actually beneficial to your skin, a 5–10-minute shower will actually benefit your skin, and when you moisturize immediately after it will be beneficial. The practices in Dermatology for children with acute flares of eczema are actually often "wet wraps," where cloths are saturated with water and then wrapped over the affected areas for 15 minutes, then medications are applied. The water can actually help to hydrate the skin.

2. Do you Lather up really well with soap?

I ask it this way, so if you happen to be guilty of scrubbing like there is a soap commercial "shoot" going on in your bathroom every day you will be more likely to be honest about your starring role. I find that men, by a large majority, are the more likely to scrub very well in the shower . . . and then they don't moisturize, it's just not a "manly" thing to do. And of course, I will tease a bit on that. But, do we really need to be scrubbing with soap everywhere this way, every day? My response may seem basic, and well, sound pretty *dirty*, but it is common sense that has been passed on to me by the great people in my career. I would ask you the question then, how did everybody do it before us? You know, before all the heated running water, before all the commercial soap? Yeah, you know, everyone that has essentially come on this planet before us. My point isn't that we should not be bathing, nor is it that we should not be using soap. It is important to wash daily all the areas that truly need soap and lathering . . . underarms/groin.

The business end of skincare sometimes gets in

the way of common sense. "They" want to sell you soap and creams, and sell this idea of being germ free. Just look at what happened in the 50s with formula and breast feeding, they told all these young women that formula was superior to breast milk, and anyone who breastfed was looked upon as a cave person. We have to look past what is being told to us sometimes, and think for ourselves. I come across as an unclean person, in this book, and probably to my patients, but I gain their trust when they start to think it through, and when their skin starts to feel better than ever.

3. Are you using a wash cloth or a sponge?

The answer to this is sometimes just hands, or a loofa, soft sponge or washcloths. I secretly love to hear that you are using something to scrub, because I actually really enjoy explaining the importance of avoiding such practices, and this is partly why I actually love Dermatology. Aside from my obvious distaste for the overuse of soap, the use of something abrasive is one of the worst things you can do for your skin. Let me explain why . . . It is natural to think that exfoliating with something would be good for your skin, you know, scrape off the dead skin, the germs, the grease, etc. Well, let me go ahead and tear all that apart. Firstly, these "fomites" are a breeding ground for bacteria and fungus and dead skin cells, so how do you like that idea of scrubbing all that all over your body. Doesn't sound to appealing, right? Well, you may be one of those patients that tells me you are using a clean cloth every day, and that may even be the case, but it is probably not the hygienic part of the use of a washcloth that really isn't good for skin, it is the fact that it is abrasive. You may be using the softest cloth ever, but it is still going to be stripping off a layer of dead skin cells and oils on the skin. Now, your skin as I said is a lot smarter than you or me, and it has worked very hard to make this "brick and mortar" basket weave-like structure with many layers. The layers of protection prevent moisture loss, and create a physical barrier preventing infection with bacteria, fungi and viruses.

When you wash with an abrasive cloth or sponge you are making thousands of microscopic breaks in the skin, very superficial, but they are enough to assist in the drying out of your skin and potential vulnerability for you to pick up a germ. This is proven in practice, children with dry skin and eczema tend to get viral warts more easily, and will have numerous warts, and children with eczema tend to get bacterial impetigo more easily and herpes infections just to name a few. So, it is not just by opinion that this is so important.

I try to make people understand by giving them a scenario, where you are taking care of this little baby, and the baby has a skin condition, say horrible eczema, now would you take that wash cloth with soap and lather this baby? Even where the skin problem sites are, the answer is everyone kind of laughs, looks sheepish, and says no. Then I ask, so why would we want to do that with your skin? I want you to take care of your skin as you would baby's skin.

4. What type of cleanser are you using?

I know people try to tell me that the soap they are using is mild, that it says sensitive skin, heck it even says moisturizing, and to top it all off it is Dermatologist approved. Soap is soap and it is still going to pull the natural oils from your skin, and these oils are meant to be there, our skin is smarter than we are. It is so hard for your skin to keep up with a regimen like that, even if you moisturize it doesn't fully replace what has been lost. We are so used to being "squeaky" clean, but this is not a good thing, especially if you are suffering from chronic dry skin, get itchy for unknown reasons, or have eczema or psoriasis. I am not against being clean, we should be, that is the beauty of the 21st century, but we should be with moderation.

Use an oil cleanser! Be wary of cleansers that say "gentle" because these also will behave like soap even if they are marketed otherwise. Not showering more than once daily is also helpful. Cleansers may be labeled as very mild, but what I recommend the most is an oil cleanser. Oil cleansers remove the sweat and grime from our skin but allows your skins to maintain its natural oils.

I also urge you to avoid the regular use of antibacterial soaps, unless directed by your dermatologist, otherwise, stop trying to get rid of bacteria with these. If you have a skin condition such as eczema and have been instructed to reduce the bacterial load on the skin, you can consider the use of weekly bleach baths. It sounds extreme byThe ratio of bleach to water is so small that it is similar to pool water, and will not hurt your skin or burn. The amount is ½ cup bleach to a half-filled tub, or if for a child in a bath basin it is 1 tablespoon or capful. What the bleach bath will help to do is really decrease the bacteria on the skin, and help reduce flaring of the eczema and prevent superinfection of any skin lesions. This is accomplished without drying skin, you need not stay in the water more than 5–10 minutes. Studies have shown this method to be successful at preventing eczema flares in the patients who follow this.

It is actually my belief that there is a natural balance to skin, and to the flora that exists on every square inch of our skin. I like to think of it as warring colonies, they keep each other under control because they are constantly at war. For example, if you are constantly using hand sanitizer, and have an extremely low bacterial load you will be giving yourself the opportunity to become heavily colonized by a harmful type of bacteria simply because there is no competition. This has been shown in neonatal intensive care units, they observed that neonates actually had better survival rates when they were given skin-to-skin contact with their mothers, it has been coined "kangarooing." The principle is the same, the baby becomes colonized by the healthy balance of bacteria by the mother, instead of being left in a sterile environment and vulnerable to picking up a nasty bug in the hospital. It ties into what I said above, if everyone was able to survive on this planet up until now, we must agree that there is something to be said about staying natural when possible.

5. When you are done, do you moisturize?

It is very important to moisturize after the shower! This is the absolute best time to seal in hydration because our skin absorbs it so much better. After a shower the skin has retained water from bathing, and the application of a cream will help to maintain the hydration. Creams and lotions will also penetrate skin better after it has been wet, allowing for even better moisturizing power. All the more reason to moisturize right after your shower.

6. Do you finish your skincare with a body oil?

To seal in these layers of moisture and cream completing the process with a little oil works very well. The oil works to create a water barrier and when using a natural oil such as almond oil, rich in vitamin E and antioxidants it will also promote youthful healthy skin. This works best right after the shower when the skin is still a little damp, and you can gently towel dry after. This is especially popular for those who prefer to skip the moisturizer and go straight from showering to applying an oil. Some people just don't like to apply creams and would prefer using only oils. This can work great, as long as you do not have very dry skin, which usually responds best to both the application of a cream and a finishing layer of oil. For the winter months in particular it is a good practice to layer moisturizers and oils after the shower to protect your skin.

CHAPTER

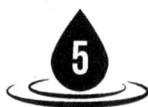

5

"Oils We Love"

Chronically dry skin can seem resistant to the "best" cleansers and richest of moisturizers. When the focus is shifted on how we bathe, with a reduction of cleanser use on areas that do not require the use of soaps, we can begin to see the change in skin quality. It can take 2–3 weeks of changing the way that one is bathing prior to seeing the improvement in overall skin hydration and the health of the outer layers of skin.

Once we move past the notion of using soaps on essential parts of the body first, then we can talk about moisturizing and, most importantly, the "sealing" of moisturizers with the use of oils. The finishing

oil layer can help to maintain the level of skin hydration by creating a water barrier that prevents the skin from drying out while retaining the benefit of the moisturizer for longer periods of time, as well.

Natural oils provide abundant resources of nutrients, antioxidants, and also provide a rich balance of long- and short-chain fatty acids that can help promote a healthier environment for skin cells and the overall bacterial biome that exists on all of our skin. It is important to have a healthy colonization of bacteria on our skin, especially when treating skin conditions such as eczema, acne, rosace, or psoriasis that we most commonly see in dermatology.

The so called "good" bacteria actually help to reduce the infective properties of certain bacteria, making it more challenging for a pathogen to survive and cause imbalance and skin infection. The importance of healthy bacteria, as discussed, is recognized in neonatal care; mothers are encouraged to have skin-to-skin contact with their newborn to help promote the colonization of healthy bacteria to help improve the health and survival of the baby. Balance is everything when it comes to taking care of your skin, and at the end of the day you have to use your judgment and common sense when taking care of your skin.

The oils we love to use in our Simply Oil collection for the face and body are carefully selected for their unique properties and ability to promote healthy glowing skin without being too rich or heavy. We want to deliver the most potent benefits and results without encouraging clogged pores. Another important point when we are formulating our face oils is to use oils that are not heavily processed. Oils can be derived from natural sources via several methods. The first and best method is called cold pressing. In simple terms, the plant or seed/nut is squeezed under high pressure to extract the natural oils. The oils expressed with this "cold press" approach have the highest content of antioxidants and natural beneficial compounds. The second press is often performed under high heat, which destructs many of these delicate compounds rendering unwanted changes in the oil product.

Other ways of extracting oils include the use of chemicals to refine and withdraw the product from its source, and this can lead to trace amounts of chemicals that we do not want to put on our skin. Therefore, when sourcing oils, it is in our best interest to use minimally processed oils that are cold pressed and unrefined. For example, we can talk about coconut oil. Coconut oil, in its most natural state, is solid at room temperature and has a balance of short and long fatty acids that have natural antimicrobial properties. When coconut oil becomes refined, these beneficial properties are lost, and the oil is no longer solid at room temperature and is liquid. The liquid coconut oil may be easier to use in some instances, but it will not provide the other health benefits that are so special.

There are some oils that are best used for the management of dry skin on the face and neck and then there are many others that work best for dry skin on the body. The choice of oil will also vary depending on the skin issues being addressed and location. The most important thing to know is that a little truly does go a long way. Many people are turned off of the idea of using oils in skincare, and this is perhaps because the experiences that they have had involved the use of way too much oil. It is really only a little that is needed in order to provide the health benefits and maintain moisture levels. For example, a full face requires no more that 2–3 drops of oil. You can use oils which are mostly for the face, which include rose hip seed oil, jojoba oil, marula oil, apricot seed oil, and grapeseed oil.

In recent years, we have seen a paradigm shift from all oil-free products to the inclusion of oils in cleansers, creams, and serums. This shift in how we're taking care of skin has a lot to do with how our skin barrier functions and the understanding that both the natural oils made by our skin and oils derived from nature are beneficial to maintaining hydrated, soft, healthy skin. The added benefit to using oils is some also have properties that can help rejuvenate skin and reverse signs of aging.

OILS WE LOVE
Apricot Seed Oil

We love apricot seed oil for its lightweight feel and heavyweight impact on skin protection and rejuvenation. It is a mildly scented golden oil that is cold pressed from the kernels of apricots. They are rich in phyto-nutrients and help to smooth the appearance of wrinkles. The oil can be helpful for dry skin and eczema and does not typically clog pores, making it a great option for most skin types.

It is rich in skin healthy fatty acids, oleic and linoleic acids that help moisturize and protect more mature skin. Apricot seed oil is very hydrating and promotes skin softness. Apricot seed oil also contains vitamin C and E, which help promote bright even skin tones and promote collagen production.

Marula Oil

Marula oil is unique for its high oleic acid content, with an average up to 78%. It is derived from the fruit of a tree native to South Africa, *Sclerocarya Birrea*. Marula oil is also high in glutamic acid and L-arginine, which have anti-aging properties and help promote skin hydration levels. Marula oil is high in antioxidants, helping to protect skin against free radicals and oxidative damage.

Argan Oil

Argan oil is derived from kernels that grow on argan trees that are native to Morocco. It is used widely in skin care, hair care, and cosmetics. It is known for its anti-aging properties, anti-oxidant activity, and helps to keep skin smooth and maintain hydration. It can also be helpful in the skin care of those treating acne.

Grapeseed Oil

Grapeseed oil is derived from the tiny seeds from grapes, pressing the seeds helps to extract the fruits oil. Oily skin and acne benefit from the use of grape seed oil for its lightweight emollient and non-pore clogging ability. It is high in antioxidants and, in addition to its moisturizing properties, it is also anti-inflammatory. It has naturally occurring vitamin C and E, which help to brighten skin tone and protect from photodamage and oxidative stress.

Castor Oil

One oil I read about a lot that can help with dark circles in castor oil—what in this oil can help lighten skin and improve the look of the under-eye area?

Castor oil has been shown to have potent antioxidant activity, and among other health benefits is its role in hemagglutination. This property can help resolve the purplish discoloration from blood vessels in the delicate skin under the eyes.

Rosemary Oil

To help thinning hair, can you talk about the benefits of rosemary oil? I've read that it can increase blood flow and bring oxygen and nutrients to hair follicles. How does this help thin hair? Rosemary oil has been said, throughout history, to be beneficial for hair regrowth. We know it is antioxidant rich. In 2015, a study of 100 patients, where 50 people were assigned topical rosemary oil and the other 50 topical minoxidil, they found that at the 6-month marker both groups had significant regrowth of hair.

Virgin Coconut Oil

Are there any other oils you would recommend for skin or hair and how do they work? Any recommendations for dry skin?

Virgin coconut oil is a favorite of mine. It has antioxidants, and natural antimicrobial properties. It is great for cradle cap, psoriasis, seborrheic dermatitis, eczema, and dry skin. Many patients are able to regain control over their skin conditions with regular use of virgin coconut oil. For dry skin, I recommend moisturizing first then sealing with a fine layer of virgin coconut oil.

Rosehip Seed Oil

Rosehip oil is another favorite of mine. It has great anti-inflammatory properties and works well to reduce the appearance of fine lines and wrinkles; it also works well on sensitive skin and rosacea prone skin.

6

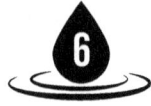

"Rosacea and Acne"

Rosacea and acne are incredibly common and interesting skin conditions that at some point will affect up to 80% of us. So many people ask me what causes acne or what causes rosacea. I don't really have a clear answer for what causes these conditions. I wish I did. And, to my knowledge, nobody really has the answer. We have tons of research; we have tons of therapies, regimens, and diet modifications, but we don't really have an answer. This is really because there is no one single answer, at least not yet, that has been uncovered. I consider rosacea and acne to be a reactive type of skin conditions that are really due to a combination of factors, which include genetics, environment, stress, topical factors, hormones, and nutritional factors. So, I don't have a silver bullet to help treat these conditions, or an aha moment that we can pinpoint what the causes for any particular patient that is struggling with these conditions. What I do like to do, though, in my daily practice—and this is from experience, trial and error, and extensive reading—is to approach it from all these different angles that I have mentioned. When you have a multi-angle approach, you will have the best outcomes, which are sustainable and more consistent. When you are targeting the root cause of a condition, you'll have a better success rate and the overall health of the patient will improve.

Oils play a role in the management of rosacea and acne. For many people, the stigma of oils that they have read about or heard about from others prevents them from maintaining a healthy skin barrier. And what is true for both of these conditions is a healthy skin barrier is necessary to maintain and promote healing and reduce "flareups" of their conditions. Many people who struggle with skin conditions such as rosacea and acne instinctively feel that their skin is breaking out because it's not clean or they have germs on their skin. So, in turn, they extensively clean their skin with complicated skin care regimens that often interrupt their skin barrier, and lead to damaged areas that are prone to irritation from chemicals in the environment and can become a nidus for infection. When the skin barrier is not intact, it cannot tolerate application of many skin care products and prescription topical medications.

For rosacea, from my top-to-bottom approach, usually I'll first look into what the person has been eating and what kind of lifestyle they have. And I will educate them as to the importance of a low inflammatory diet, explain that there's excess that will not be only from a cream or only from a prescription, and it really has to be a comprehensive approach. Many patients who struggle with rosacea will also have an intolerance to gluten and sometimes dairy. Gluten is a well-known inflammatory protein and dairy contains whey protein, which is also known for being inflammatory. Reducing or eliminating gluten and dairy, specifically cow's milk, can support better clearance and more consistent outcomes in rosacea. I get a lot of push back from patients who do not want to make the effort to change their diet. It seems an insurmountable task. They can't imagine their life without a loaf of Italian bread at the dinner table and a bowl of pasta. And what I say to that patient or person is take it one day at a time, find smart substitutions for things that you love. They make excellent brown rice pasta that can stay al dente and not turn into mush. It does exist and you can find it. And, over time, somebody who's been accustomed to eating bread every day of their life will slowly learn not to eat bread every meal and still feel satisfied. I wouldn't harp on this if I didn't, in practice, see that it made such a big difference in the patients who cut it out of their diet. It's the truth that it can take 2 to 3 months of adhering to a low-inflammatory diet to see improvement in one's skin, but once they see it, they recognize it's from a diet change. And in many of the patients who have switched over and are doing well, they'll report that if they ate a slice of pizza or they had ice cream or bread and pasta that a good two days later they noticed that they had developed a nice flareup of the rosacea. Aside from my feelings on the topic, there are numerous research articles that actually support these findings.

What are the best supplements for acne and rosacea? Along with the idea of how important nutrition is for our skin and acne, there are several key supplements that can help keep your skin looking clear. A combination of vitamins and natural supplements can help to maintain healthy skin and nails. It is important to remember that supplements can take

8–12 weeks before significant changes are noted in our skin . . . so be patient and do not give up. In my office, I consult patients on diet, supplements, skin care, and will also prescribe topical and oral therapies as adjuncts to treatment, but I first make a note to stress the importance of diet and supplements.

I will go over which supplements work best, and how to pick which ones for your skin. Rosacea and acne have a lot of overlap when it comes to oral supplements. For hormonal acne, I have a few recommendations that are specific for women. If you have a health condition or are taking medications, always speak with your doctor before starting a new supplement.

VITAMIN A

This power vitamin works on much more than just vision, it is integral to our immune function and plays a powerful role in skin, hair, and nails. In fact, the treatment known as Accutane is essentially a synthetic form of vitamin A, so it would make sense that supplementation with vitamin A would be of benefit to your skin. (However, if already taking Accutane, do not take vitamin A supplements). A daily dose of 5.000 I.U. in an oil capsule, in the retinol form, I find is most beneficial. Take with a fatty meal, such as dinner.

NIACINAMIDE (VITAMIN B3)

This vitamin has a potent anti-inflammatory effect on the skin, in addition to its importance in maintaining the barrier function of our skin. Niacinamide is particularly helpful for *both* acne and rosacea. The recommended dosage is 500–800mg twice daily. Unlike Niacin, Niacinamide should not cause redness or flushing of the skin.

ZINC

There are many studies that have shown the benefit of taking zinc daily in the reduction of acne and rosacea. Zinc is essential to the proper function of our skin and can be found in many foods, such as pumpkin seeds, oysters, and beef. Zinc picolinate or chelated zinc may have better absorption and effect than zinc gluconate. The general recommended dose is 50mg per day. This will not only help rosacea and acne, but will probably prevent or ease the common cold. Make sure to take zinc with food to prevent stomach upset.

BORAGE OIL AND EVENING PRIMROSE OIL

If you have never heard of either of these oils, they are widely used for the treatment of menopausal symptoms, PMS, and work great for the hormonal component of acne. These oils are derived from plants and are high in anti-inflammatory fatty acids. They are precursors to the production of our own hormones; this can help to stabilize imbalances. Many patients swear by this for their acne, and I am often recommending this for hormonal acne. Often hormonal acne will be noted in the beard distribution, along the jawline, lower cheeks, and upper neck area, but can also include the chest and back.

PROBIOTICS

Our gut flora and digestive tracts have a strong impact on acne and rosacea, as well. It may sound like a lot of supplements, but maintaining a healthy gut should not be overlooked for its importance. A natural way to increase your intake of good bacteria is to eat fermented foods such as sauerkraut and kimchi (these are non-dairy recommendations).

SPEARMINT TEA

No kidding. Studies have shown that 1 cup twice daily reduced hormonal acne and even facial hair in women. With a mild mint flavor, this tea is very pleasant. To sweeten it, try a teaspoon of raw honey (also so good for you).

GREEN TEA

The powerful green tea polyphenols found in this tea work well for your overall health, and are wonderful anti-oxidants that can help brighten your complexion and reduce both acne and rosacea flares.

In addition to a low inflammatory diet, taking supplements that can help reduce inflammation are also important in the treatment of rosacea and acne. Usually I will recommend zinc, niacinamide, or a multivitamin gummy that can contains these vitamins to treat acne. For acne patients who are female, I will also sometimes recommend spearmint capsules or drinking spearmint tea, 1 cup twice daily, if there appears to be a hormonal pattern to the breakouts. It is important to make sure that you don't overdo it with any vitamins. Always check other supplements that you're taking to make sure that you're not overdoing anything and taking more than the daily recommended amount of any particular vitamin. Women who are perimenopausal may also benefit from taking evening primrose oil, which is an oral supplement that can help bring back balance and help reduce flareups, and I have seen improvement with this supplement as well for some patients.

Have you tried every over-the-counter/prescription for acne and still can't seem to stop those pimples from appearing every other day? You are definitely not alone, and this is something I deal with in my office every day. It is unrealistic to believe that all acne will improve with just topical creams and cleansers. This particularly rings true for those of you out there who have hormonal acne . . . a high number of you indeed. I will go over my general recommendations that can dramatically improve acne naturally!

It is essential to recognize the importance of what we are putting into our bodies every day. I find that, especially for acne, in order to get consistent results and eliminate flare-ups the proper diet is key. There are several food groups in particular that contribute to acne, and what I suggest has also been confirmed through dermatologic research in patterns of acne and dietary triggers.

DAIRY

Skip the cow products. Trust me. They are loaded with hormones, even if you buy organic. Think about it, this is meant for a baby cow to become a big cow rapidly. The "Western" ideology that dairy is essential to your health and bone growth is false. The calcium in milk can easily be replaced with eating dark leafy vegetables. In fact, some of the largest populations on the planet do not include dairy in their diet . . .

and they are all doing very well. I have many patients who notice that they get flare-ups after having a dairy splurge.

To avoid dairy, that means no milk, cheese, ice cream, butter, and products that have butter in them . . . so read labels. A wonderful milk replacement is Almond Milk (try Califia, it is terrific).

REFINED CARBOHYDRATES

This is the tough one to talk about. Many people will say . . . What?! No bread?! How dare you? And, I wish that this wasn't the case, but all the research shows such strong correlations with acne and the glycemic index. This means . . . try to avoid sweets, white bread, white rice, pastas, etc. Certainly, in moderation whole grains can be well tolerated, such as brown rice and bread. However, these should *not* be the main star of your meal. Avoid the bread basket when you go out to eat, either keep the towel over the bread or even ask them to not bring bread to the table. I will often have them hold the toast when ordering an omelet, if I am out.

Anecdotally, I also have seen that a gluten-free diet can help clear the skin for many patients. **It will take 8 weeks with any change in your diet or skin**

care regimen to notice a change, so I suggest you give it a real try if you think this might help you.

Then I will usually talk about skin care, and I'll ask the patient what they are doing with their skin, what is the daily routine for that person. And I believe in a less-is-more approach, and this is to help support skin care and that skin barrier, which is essential for any skin condition the basis of your skin's health. Essentially gentle skin care works for most of these patients because they have some degree of a barrier malfunction. I would recommend a very gentle cleanser. Usually they respond very well to an oil-based cleanser, which will help to remove the grime of the day and make up without stripping the skin of their natural oils and will not leave the skin feeling dry and tight. When you use an oil based, gentle cleansers, usually these patients can tolerate the prescription medications, which are very dry, better than had they been using it so called "gentle" cleanser that really strips the skin of all these oils is drying even if marketed as being super gentle, and men for the most sensitive skin types. I've really seen a lot of patients not able to tolerate the "gentlest" cleansers on the market.

After you have washed, it's important to layer

◆

TIPS FOR WHAT TO EAT

Breakfast

The American breakfast has to be the most carb driven out there. Skip the cereal, pancakes, English muffins . . . opt for eggs, a veggie omelet, or quinoa (made oatmeal style is so yummy and nutritious for breakfast). Eggs are good for you! They had a bad reputation for many years, but we now know that they have always been good. They had interviewed one of the oldest women alive, she had just turned 117, and she eats 2 eggs a day (she eats them raw, but I am definitely not suggesting that you do!). Eggs are loaded with good proteins, Vitamin A and D.

Snacks

Try snacking on a handful of nuts, or a protein bar low in sugar. Bring Apple slices and almond butter for dipping. Try a berry smoothie, this will be filled with skin-friendly antioxidants. The key is to be prepared and ready for a healthy snack when you are on the run.

Lunch

Skip the sandwich, instead opt for a salad, or a protein (such as salmon or chicken) with vegetables. If you must have a sandwich, try using an almond or coconut flour wrap, they are gluten free, low in carbs and less inflammatory. Have some fruit with your meal. Remember, the more you make food for yourself, and buy less, the cleaner and healthier your food will be.

Dinner

Eat healthy fish such as Salmon that is rich in Omegas. Select meats that are grass fed, these meats actually produce omega fatty acids that are beneficial to your health and skin. Eat plenty of vegetables. Keep your carbs to a small amount, imagine a handful of brown rice, that is not a lot. Use olive oil and coconut oil in your cooking. Not only are they good for your skin, but using oils in your food will help keep you feeling full longer, so you will not have to snack. Up your intake of legumes, such as lentils, rich in nutrients, iron and protein; they can be both filling and delicious.

your hydration in a way that's not going to be too heavy, because we don't want to clog pores. But, usually a patient with either the condition of rosacea or acne will respond well to a hyaluronic acid serum paired with a gentle moisturizer. I recommend applying serums prior to moisturizing. Depending on how dry someone's skin is, and how they are tolerating the recommended acne medications, I will sometimes suggest that the serums and moisturizers can actually be applied prior to application of the acne medications to reduce the intensity and drying effect of the acne prescriptions. Evening skin care routines benefit with the addition of the final step of applying a few drops of a face oil. The best face oil is a combination of rosehip seed oil, marula oil, apricot seed oil, and jojoba oil. We have found it to be really good for inflammation and calming skin-condition redness and irritation. For those who have extremely dry skin and would like to use an oil like this in the morning, it can be used again. We use a proprietary blend of these oils in their most pure state, loaded with antioxidants and natural fatty acid chains that help to promote healthy skin.

In addition to the management of a patient's diet, we always discuss their skin care routines and the supplements.

7

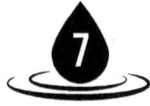

"Morning vs Night Routines"

t is important to take care of your skin. It is what we do on a regular basis that will add up over time to create the kind of results we can appreciate. It is not about how aggressive or involved a regimen is, but rather the consistent nature and adherence to a simple routine that will deliver results over the years.

I'm going to start this one by addressing the night-time routine first. This is after all the most important time for healing, repairing, and forming collagen. A recent study found that just 14% of American Men and 30% of American Women regularly use sunscreen before sun exposure, and with the coming Spring and Summer seasons (when the UV Index is at its highest[1]) we typically spend more time outdoors. It is always the time for protective measures from the sun, but it is especially important to consider how to increase your sun protection during the warmer months!

SPENDING MORE TIME IN THE SUN MEANS SPENDING MORE TIME ON SUN PROTECTION!

Here are my recommendations on how to keep your skin safest this Spring & Summer and be proactive in reducing your sun exposure:

1. Use a Physical (mineral) sunscreen on all exposed areas of the body (remember your ears!). A Physical sunscreen sits on the top of your skin and reflects harmful UVA and UVB rays. It uses mineral ingredients such as Zinc Oxide and Titanium Dioxide, which are inert and safe for all age groups, including children. Sometimes Physical sunscreens have a bad rep for being thicker and leaving a white cast, so I recommend these products that I love so much that we carry them in our office:

    — Sheer Mineral, by Simply Dermatology, is spf 50 and mineral based, it has a light formulation which is great for more oily skin types

— Elta MD Tinted Physical, a lightly tinted formula that is great for most skin types and has a soft, smooth finish

— Elta MD Body Sunscreen for the body

2. The sun's UV rays can damage your skin in as little as 15 minutes.[2] Avoid being in the sun between the hours of 10 am–4 pm (if you can) when the sun is at its highest intensity. Wear protective clothing when possible. Tighter woven fabrics offer the best protection, and there is also UPF rated sun protection clothing available. UPF is a rating for how much UV radiation is absorbed by the fabric. For instance, a UPF rating of 50 means that 1/50th of the suns UV radiation with pass through the fabric. This means it can reduce the UV rays that reach your skin by 50 times or close to 98% UV protection. So, clothing with a UPF grading of 50 works even better than regular clothing.

3. Wear a hat! About 7% of head and neck melanomas are found on the ears.[3]

4. Wear a SPF protective lip balm to protect your lips and re-apply every 2 hours, and after you drink or eat.[4]

5. Some natural oils such as Carrot or Coconut oil provide some sun protection (about SPF 4), but

they are not enough, so be sure to not rely on them solely for your sun protection.

6. Consider upping your protection from the inside out. I often recommend a daily dietary supplement containing niacinamide to help maintain your skin's ability to protect itself against the aging effects of free radicals. It helps protect skin, increases your skin's sunburn threshold, and reduces the risk of skin cancer. In fact, a diet high in antioxidants in general is a good way to increase your sun protection as well.

If you find yourself with something on your body about which you're not sure, then get a skin check from your Dermatologist. I recommend yearly skin checks just to make sure your skin is free of concern. If you find yourself with sun damage, there are also some procedures I like to do in office to help the appearance. We can reverse age spots, broken collagen, fine lines, and broken blood vessels that can all appear years after prolonged sun exposure.

1. *We know that not getting enough sleep is bad for your skin. What about getting TOO much? Is there any evidence that oversleeping can harm your skin in some way?*

During sleep, our skin has the opportunity to hydrate, repair ultraviolet sun damage, create new collagen, and many other necessary functions for daily, healthy maintenance. The experts have recommended that adults get between 7 and 9 hours of sleep daily. Does this mean that more sleep is better, though? Well, I wouldn't throw out the alarm clock just yet. There is no proven health benefit to oversleeping as a habit. In fact, habitual oversleeping has been associated with health risks such as diabetes and heart disease, and if oversleeping is not being done intentionally, it may in fact be a sign of depression, hypothyroidism, or a nutritional disorder. These conditions can show skin signs of dryness, flaking, slow healing, and may lead to similar findings in hair and nails. So, I wouldn't buy the black-out shades and force yourself to oversleep. Getting a healthy balance of both sleep and activity are essential to healthy skin.

2. *Is there any truth to the theories that higher-thread count sheets or silk pillowcases are better for your skin/hair? If so, how?*

There is no current evidence to prove or disprove this theory; however, I do believe that sleep positions play a role of importance for skin aging. If your sheets have a high thread count or are made of silk, and you still sleep on your face, it is still creating pressure and can expedite wrinkle formation. A good tip for your hair overnight is to let it loose; keeping your hair in braids or clips overnight if done routinely can put stress on your follicles and over time lead to thinning hair.

3. *Is there any type of cream (medicated or OTC) that is better to apply at night and, if so, why?*

OTC Retinol or prescription Retinoic acid creams are almost always best used at night. These creams are less effective during the day and are not stable in sunlight, so will not work as well.

4. *I read that stomach sleeping can be bad for your skin because you're pressing your face into the pillow and, over time, this pressure can cause fine lines. Is there any truth to that? (And if so, does the same go for side sleepers?)*

Sleeping on your side or stomach can promote the formation or deepening of lines and wrinkles over time. In my practice. I can often tell on which side a patient prefers to sleep because of the facial asymmetry that occurs. The side that is favored to sleep on usually has loss of volume over the cheek and deeper lines and folds around the nose and sometimes mouth and eyes. I recommend, if possible, back sleeping with 1 to 2 pillows behind your head. For patients who find themselves rolling over in their sleep, a trick that can be helpful is placing a pillow under the knees, this will usually help you to remain on your back through the night.

There are so many skin conditions that will be mitigated by a low inflammatory diet. But did you know that a low inflammatory diet can **also slow the aging process**?

Diets that are rich in antioxidants and low in sugar can help to keep our skin looking younger, as in this article[5], "Discovering the link between nutrition and skin aging" from the *Dermato-Endocrinology Journal*. Diets that have a *high glycemic index* can lead to premature glycation of collagen and other proteins in our skin, which can lead to early break down and the formation of wrinkles. Diets that are rich in antioxidants can protect our skin from photo damage, free radicals, and other oxidative stressors in the environment.

Not sure which foods on which to focus? Just

read this article in *Nature*, "The Edible Skincare Diet"; as the author says, "Eating well could be better for skin health than applying lotions and potions. But which vitamins and nutrients will yield the healthiest glow?" Read the article[6] for great nutritional advice.

Foods rich in the following vitamins and nutrients were found to be most important: C, E, D, carotenoids, β-carotene, lutein, lycopene, and omega fatty acids. A diet that is low in red meats, low in dairy products (milk, yogurt, cheese), and is rich in vegetables, fruits, dark leafy greens, nuts, and great sources of omega fatty acids such as wild salmon can provide large amounts of antioxidants, a low glycemic index, and can help to reduce inflammation in the body and skin.

It is very interesting to see the impact of a low inflammatory diet on a chronic condition such as psoriasis, rosacea or acne among other many other inflammatory conditions. Clinically, when I see a patient who has changed their diet to a low inflammatory nutrition profile, it is often reflected in their skin. I will see improvements in their acne, rosacea, or psoriasis, with more consistent and predictable outcomes and fewer flare ups. **Diet and nutrition are the most important considerations when formulating a comprehensive treatment plan for my patients.**

Unfortunately, many of us with medical backgrounds are not taught extensively on the impact of nutrition and diet on medical conditions. So due to lack of education and shortened medical visits, this can sometimes be overlooked. Research shows that it is undeniably one of the most important parts of the treatment plan for many skin conditions. A healthy diet will reflect on many different organ systems, including your skin.

8

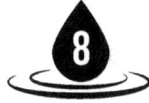

"Skin Questionnaire"

Q: *Do you think it is necessary to have different skin care routines/products based on seasonal changes?*

A: We should consider the climate when choosing what kinds of products to apply on our skin. For winter months, or drier climates, you may want to use a richer moisturizer and facial serum and cleanse with a light wash that won't over-dry your skin. In more humid and warmer months, using lighter serums and moisturizers will prevent pore clogging, and a cleanser that will help reduce sweat build up and clean pores will keep skin in better balance.

Q: *Are anti-aging moisturizers really effective? If so, which one would you recommend?*

A: Anti-aging moisturizers are definitely important as part of the skin care regimen, and usually are started in late 20s to early 30s. Simply Collection's face cream contains natural oils that help the rejuvenation process, working to improve elasticity and reverse the aging process. It is a hydrating cream that leaves skin feeling very soft.

Q: *What types of products do you swear by for dry skin (face and body)?*

A: For dry skin on the body, I prefer moisturizing and finishing with a body oil. For dry skin on the face, I recommend a hydrating hyaluronic serum followed by moisturizer and sealed with a small amount of a specialized face oil, such as Simply Dermatology's collection.

Q: *Besides wearing sunscreen, is there one skin care tip you think all women should follow at any age?*

A: Wash your face every night and make sure to cleanse make-up from your skin. This is an essential part of the skincare routine; it will prevent clogged pores and allow for skin treatments to penetrate better on the skin.

Q: *Should I change my skin care routine in the winter vs summer? Is it possible to over moisturize your face in humidity? (And how to know if you are)*

A: An optimal skin care regimen should be flexible and climate should really be taken into account when choosing the right products to use and how much to put on. We frequently discuss how to take care of skin during periods of cold weather and low humidity, but we often dismiss the management of skincare in humid climates. High humidity can provide a moisture-rich environment for your skin, but can be challenging for patients with oily skin types and for those with acne-prone skin. The extra hydration on the skin and lack of evaporation can lead to a residue build up on the skin that can result in clogged pores. It can also cause makeup to run and look shiny or dewy.

I often recommend changing up creams that were being used in colder and drier climates and switching to lighter lotions or serums, which are non-comedogenic. A good example of a very nice light lotion with SPF 30 is Cerave AM Lotion. The amount that should be applied will be different for each person. You want to have enough so that the lotion easily rubs into the skin and disappears. Powder makeup or

◆

TOP 7 TIPS FOR DRY
SKIN IN WINTER!

Winter is one of the most trying times for many of my patients when it comes to their skin care routine. It really comes down to the combination of such stressors as low humidity, high heat from being indoors, and the cold outdoor elements like the frigid winter wind that really dry out our skin.

To combat all of this, though, there are a few things on which we can focus specifically during these months:

1. Soap up the right way. The first thing on which to focus is making use of gentle skin care. Target soap on the parts of the body that truly needs washing and avoid lathering it all over the body. The reason this approach is effective, especially during the winter, is because when soap is applied to our skin, it washes away our natural oils that our skin needs!

2. Use an oil cleanser! Be wary of cleansers that say "gentle" because these also will behave like soap even if they are marketed otherwise. Not showering more than once daily is also helpful. Cleansers such as Cerave or Cetaphil are very mild, but what I recommend the most is an oil cleanser. Oil cleansers remove the sweat and grime from our skin but allows your skins to maintain its natural oils.

3. Don't over wash! Showers should be brief, 5 minutes, warm but not hot water, and never shower more than once daily. Cleanliness is important, but it is not good to over wash. Washing twice daily can make it really difficult for our skin to keep up with maintaining natural oil levels.

4. Ditch the loofah. When washing it really is best to use your hands. Washing with a cloth or sponge will strip your skin of the supportive outer layers, these layers are working hard to retain moisture and provide a healthy barrier protecting you from the environment.

5. Moisturize after the shower! This is the abso-lute best time to seal in hydration because our skin absorbs it much better.

6. Apply an after-shower oil! A really great addition to this winter skin care routine is sealing all of that great hydration in with an oil, like Simply Dermatology's Simply Body Oil, rich in Sweet almond oil (only if there is no allergy), which is high in Vitamin E and other antioxidants.

7. Humidify your environment. This is espe-cially helpful in your bedroom, maintaining the humidity levels can help maintain skin hydration for those who suffer from eczema and severe dry skin.

light lotion-based makeup that is oil free will perform well in high humidity. A good finishing makeup setting spray can be used to help prevent makeup from running as well.

ACNE, PSORIASIS, ECZEMA, ROSACEA

Q: *In general, what does the colder temperatures do to our skin?*

A: There are several reasons for why our skin suffers and many skin conditions worsen during colder months. Cold air has a reduced ability to hold moisture, which leads to dry skin. The ideal indoor humidity should be held at 30–50%, and with heating systems this can drop down to as low as 15% in the winter. Outside our skin has to deal with low temperatures and chilling winds that result in wind burn.

Q: *Can you please offer 3 tips each (aside from seeing your derma and possibly getting a prescription) on how readers can treat these 4 conditions: acne, psoriasis, eczema and rosacea.*

1. Acne

In the winter, moisturizing is key to maintain clear skin. Proper hydration is necessary to maintain a healthy skin barrier, and will also allow skin to tolerate the topical acne cleansers and treatments being used.

Do not over wash. Wash your face no more than twice daily, and you may want to switch to a gentler cleanser, or even use an oil-based wash over the winter months to spare your skin the natural oils.

Switch to a better moisturizer for your skin if you are drying out. A more hydrating and richer moisturizer may be necessary during these colder drier months. Make sure the product is labeled "non-comedogenic."

2. Psoriasis

Do not bathe more than once daily, use a gentle cleanser, and take 5-minute *warm* showers.

Moisturize regularly, twice daily is recommended, and directly after the shower is the best time to apply for best absorption.

Take a vitamin D supplement every day. During the winter you will be getting less natural sunlight, and vitamin D has been shown to be important in reducing psoriatic flares.

3. Eczema

Humidify your home, especially your bedroom, to help maintain skin hydration. This will help reduce eczema flares.

Switch to a rich moisturizing cream that contains ceramides, which will help maintain the barrier and help repair skin. Apply generously twice daily.

Avoid over washing, bathe only once daily with a mild cleanser. Only use your hands, no sponges or wash cloths.

4. Rosacea

Protect your skin from the elements, if outside for prolonged periods in the cold make sure to wear a scarf to cover your lower face. The cold dry wind can be a big trigger for a rosacea flare.

Warm up with a cup of green tea during your day or take a green tea supplement if you are sensitive to hot beverages. The antioxidant effect of green tea can help reduce inflammation and may reduce flares if taken regularly.

Make sure to use a cream in the morning with SPF 30 or higher. During the colder months we often forget about the role of the sun in triggering flares, and ultraviolet rays reflect off snow and a sun burn is even possible this time of year if outside and unprotected.

◆

TOP TIPS FOR IMPROVING THE HEALTH OF YOUR NAILS

BRITTLE NAILS: Goodbye short brittle nails! Here are the best 5 tips to improve the health of your nails!

Nails that easily break, split, refuse to grow, and appear ridged are a common issue. Many times, this can be caused or either worsened by certain practices: exposure to harsh soaps and water numerous times per day, frequent use of nail polish and polish removers, alcohol-based hand sanitizers, and rarely can be a sign of an underactive thyroid or other systemic deficiency or condition. If you have such other symptoms as dry brittle hair, dry skin, lethargy, or weight-gain, you should see your dermatologist for an evaluation and work-up to rule out hypothyroidism.

Nails grow very slowly and it can take on average 3 months to see improvement in nail growth if positive changes in the daily routine are made.

Here is a list of 5 recommendations to help your nails:

1. Take daily Biotin 5,000mcg/day, this supplement has been shown to help nails grow healthier
2. Use gentle cleansers to wash hands; stop alcohol-based hand sanitizers, and polish removers.
3. Moisturize your hands several times throughout the day
4. Apply a cuticle oil before bedtime. Rosehip oil, Coconut oil, or Argan oil all work well!
5. If no improvement is noticed, consider seeing your Dermatologist. Your doctor may want to prescribe a topical medication, Genadur, for nails; it is applied to nails twice daily. Genadur is an FDA-approved prescribed medication that can make a big difference in nails that otherwise won't improve.

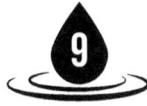

"Stories of Inspiration"

THE "CHRISTOPH WALTZ" PATIENT

I would like to share a few inspiring patient stories that have greatly impacted my own life. There are many times in which I really feel truly privileged to be in the presence of some of the most amazing people, who are so positive and really create such a strong narrative for themselves on how they view their lives and show us how just looking at something in your life, whether it's a challenge or an illness any kind of struggle, can be approached in such different ways, depending on your outlook. This ability to control your narrative really does seem like it is common sense and is obvious, but all I can say is I don't think for myself that it is that obvious and maybe for some people it comes more naturally. I think, for a lot of us, we need to be reminded to really tell ourselves a better narrative about our lives, and only good things come from what I've seen. I know this is a book about oils and skin care, but being a skin-care specialist and working with so many different people, I do want to share some of the most delicate and at the same time strong moments in my career with a few patients who actually inspired me as a human being, as a practitioner, as a mother, as a wife, and as a person.

This first patient that I want to talk about is a gentleman who was coming in for many visits over the course of two years. He was coming with his daughter and when I met them, she was around 14 years old. She was coming for the treatment of cystic acne that was hormonal and we ended up treating her with Accutane, which required monthly visit over the course of six months. The father and daughter were super charming, just really nice people and very pleasant on all of their visits. We developed a nice friendship, a wonderful patient-physician relationship, and I felt very warmly toward them; and I think that they felt the same as well. At one point, the daughter wanted to have a second ear piercing. Because she

was only 14 and that I'm not an ear-piercing estab-
lishment, even though I do repair ear piercings and I
do re-pierce ears, I wanted to give them a minute to
think about it before she went ahead and did that.
Essentially, I didn't want to be the person to pierce
her ears and then you know, years from now, she
remembers it and she regrets doing it. To preface
what the father was like, just picture the character
played by Christoph Waltz in the movie *Inglorious
Bastards*. He was also of Austrian descent and looked
and sounded just like Christoph Waltz. He was a super
pleasant guy and seemed like a pretty cool dad, and I
said, "Why don't you take a little time to think about
getting the ear piercing," . . . "you know, would you
mind if you thought about it for a month, before your
finally decide to get the second piercing? And if you
still do, I will be happy to perform the piercing for
you. I don't want you to have any regrets." Fast forward two months: they come back and he said, "I
thought about what you said, we talked it over, and
we decided we want to do those earrings still." So,
we went ahead and pierced her ears and that turned
out great.

On a subsequent visit, the father was telling me
he wanted to bring his wife for a skin exam. I had at
this point never met her, and they had never really

mentioned her. I never really thought about why she wasn't there for any of the daughter's visits and I said, that's great, definitely bring her and she's probably due for a full skin exam. The next time I saw them was a few months later for the skin exam with his wife. I had no idea that she had a disability; she was wheelchair-bound due to an autoimmune disease that made it very difficult for her to walk. She was a young, beautiful woman and she must've been only in her mid-40s. It was a little surprising because I just wasn't expecting for the wife to have a disability like that and when I did her skin exam, I reached a point where I needed her to stand up so I could examine her legs. I asked her gently if she was able to stand up so I could examine her legs. Her husband came up to her and helped her stand up. It was such a tender moment in a very vulnerable situation. He supported her in the exam room while she put this paper-thin exam gown on, and she can't stand up on her own so he has to help her. He is standing there close in front of her and she's got her arms draped around his neck to hold for support and he says, "Look, we are dancing." And that moment has stayed with me all these years later; that moment is everything. I will never forget seeing such devotion, such utter genuine love. This man took an awkward moment for anybody and made it a sweet tender moment for her. He made it fun and playful. He is just an amazing person and I think I only wish I could aspire to be positive and as strong as someone like him. Never once did he seem like he didn't want to be there for all those visits with his daughter, never once did he complain about the long wait times. It was like a scene out of a movie, so sweet. I don't know that I would be half as strong as he was and as unabashed.

THE "CLINT EASTWOOD" PATIENT

Doing the kind of work that I do, I get to see young people, newborns, people in their acne phases, people in their skin-cancer phases, all different stages of life. Being a Dermatologist, it is a real privilege getting to treat all these different people who really need our help. Now and then you just meet somebody with whom you really connect and they inspire you; they become like family after years and years of seeing somebody. For instance, I have a patient that I have known for over 10 years. And before you realize it, you've met almost everybody in their family. When a patient like this comes in for a visit, it is not like a typical patient visit, it's like seeing an old friend.

Well, this "old friend," if you try to imagine somebody around 80 years old and who looks like Clint

Eastwood, then you can imagine this patient. This guy, over the span of 10 years, has said some of the best lines I've ever heard. My medical assistant and I have had some of the best conversations with this gentleman through the years and he is always such a great source of wisdom and inspiration with how he views life and what he tells himself. What I mean by what he tells himself is better explained with examples of some of the funny stuff that he has said that has made us kind of really look back at ourselves and question what is really important. He taught us, without even trying, how you can talk to yourself to make yourself see things in a better light, in a more positive light.

On one of his visits, we were complaining about the weather, winter was coming, and my assistant and I had a visit with "Clint." Try to imagine the voice of Suzie from *Marvelous Ms. Maizel* and the voice of Janice from *Seinfeld*, the combination of these two make the voice of my lovely medical assistant, she should have had a job in show biz. So, during one of our visits. we were talking with this "Clint Eastwood" gentleman and we're complaining about the winter and we're saying this weekend it's going to snow a lot and blah blah and who wants to shovel! Well, "Clint" does not agree, and you know what he said, he said,

"I don't mind the snow, it's OK, I kind of like It. I ask myself how many more times do we have to shovel snow? How many more chances do I get?" And he elaborated by saying, "I even feel that way about the fall. I don't mind raking the leaves I figure how many more times do I have left to rake leaves?"

My assistant and I have talked about this moment so many times because he's right, what are we to complain about? We're alive, the seasons are changing, there's so much to appreciate, and no reason to complain all the time.

There was another time he was in the office and we somehow came onto the topic of getting older and what it's like to get old. And he was saying that, for him, in getting older he found that one of the biggest concerns is the feeling of not being needed by others, of not feeling necessary, and not having purpose. He was saying that's why he likes to keep the trailer for his car, in case anybody needs him, even if the grandkids need something moved, they call him and he loves that. He said, "I love being helpful, and being useful."

I don't know too many people who like to be helpful like that. It's just a beautiful way of looking at life and not complaining, only wanting to be busy and staying positive. It has been a long time that I have known him over the course of these 10 years. During a more recent visit, he was explaining to me and one of my wonderful assistants that his wife is starting to lose her memory and that she's been diagnosed with early-stage dementia. He was saying that he was vaccinated with the coronavirus vaccine first because they could only get one appointment, and it was better that he goes first because if something happened to him who's going to take care of her. He mentioned that she had asked that day about 17 times if it was her doctor's appointment today and he said he had to tell her, "No dear, it is my visit I'm seeing the doctor today."

Hearing this, I felt so bad for them and their family, and I wanted to express my sympathy for what he was going through as a friend and I told him, "I am so sorry this must be so hard for you." My own grandmother was afflicted with Alzheimer's and my husband's grandfather also had Alzheimer's, so it is close to home for us. For these reasons, I truly can connect and I try to understand to some degree what they are going through. His reply was pretty surprising. He said, "Oh no, this isn't hard for me; you see I'm in love with her. I don't just love her; I am *in* love with her and when you're in love with somebody these kinds of things are not hard." When he said that, I lost it, I held my breath; it was so powerful. His display of strength, reserve, and his ability to stay positive under these circumstances created an emotional, poignant moment, to the point that my assistant had to leave the room because she didn't want to cry in front of him. This guy was the ultimate man in a world where being manly doesn't have to be, you know, it doesn't have to be a chauvinistic thing. He was being strong and he was being true to his love for her. I mean all of us would want someone to say something like this about us if we were sick, I mean, would you be that person if you had somebody get super sick around you? Would you say that about your spouse or your significant other?

I would like to hope and think that we would all be strong and passionate like that, but I don't know for sure. I mean, I don't think that your average person is this strong that they wouldn't complain or they wouldn't be scared or concerned. But maybe he is, and this is how you know he does. He comes from a different school of thought. I know a lot of people from the older generations are kind of made of something a little tougher than the rest of us, and when they need to be strong, they're just really strong. But he is an inspiration. When he said "I am in love with her and when you're in love with somebody this is not hard," it continues to inspire me every day. I have shared this the story to many people who are struggling and going through something difficult in their lives. We all need to have a little inner Clint Eastwood, to charge through our days and through our darkest moments with grace and strength, and most importantly love.

THE HARD-OF-HEARING CHAMPION

I had another patient who was also just amazing, in the sense that she was a warrior champion, the kind of woman who doesn't complain when things get tough, the kind of woman who takes care of her husband when she herself is 85 years old and incredibly hard of hearing. She was taking care of her 88-year-old husband who had severe late-stage Parkinson's and was wheelchair-bound. This woman was coming in for frequent visits over the course of 2 years and has since passed away. But it was an honor to know her and an honor to take care of her, to be her and her husband's Dermatologist. They were coming for skin exams and she would bring him in for many small, and when I say small, most other people would consider these to be small skin rashes or irritations in the diaper area that he would get because he was incontinent. It was not easy for them to come for

their visits. This was a man who understood everything but couldn't speak and required a wheelchair,
required an ambulance to bring him to the office visits and she wasn't in any shape to do all these things
for him. So, this woman was like a saint. She would
bring him in and take care of him in a way that I
haven't seen anybody take care of their loved ones.

She was tireless, she was vigilant in his care. She
would bring the guy and open up the diaper and she
was hard of hearing so we had to speak loudly (a
borderline shout) for her to understand us and she'd
be yelling back, but she had not one lazy bone in her
body, bringing him in and taking care of him better
than somebody even would take care of a baby. And
that, that is love, that is devotion, that is something
that you don't see you too often these days. I don't
know that these younger generations or my generation even would be as devoted or selfless as this
woman was and it was an honor to be their doctor.
And she also has inspired me personally in such a
strong way throughout all the years that I'm practicing it. I'll never forget her.

Some of the cutest patients that I've had are in
their later years of life, are still in love with each other,
and some even cut each other's hair. They come to
all their visits together and they finish each other's

sentences and they can make fun of each other and laugh at each other. I just find them to be the cutest and there's something to be said about these older generations come from a different time. . . . Where people for whatever reason were a little bit more family oriented, a little bit more giving.

You really do have a lot of power in your words and in your actions with how you treat and how you take care of those around you, whether it's your spouse or your children or your coworkers and friends. Being that strong, positive, honorable person takes a lot of strength, but it's a beautiful thing that affects those around you and inspires other people to be like you. In some ways, the office visit can be therapy for both the practitioner and the patient and it's a time for learning. and I've learned so much from all the people that I have met over the years and continue to meet. I try to always remember why I'm doing what I do, and I try to do pass these positive messages along. I do practice dermatology and it's not psychology or psychiatry, but there is so much psychology that goes into treating skin conditions and I usually will pass forward the wisdom I collect along the way. Hopefully, it may become helpful to you as it has been very helpful to me.

◆

GENERAL SKIN CARE PLAN FOR THE AM/PM

The order of application will impact how well the active ingredients will actually work. Generally, you should be applying serums, followed by moisturizers, and finally oils.

Morning Routine

Cleanse

Vitamin C, E ferulic serum

Moisturize

SPF

Evening Routine

Cleanse

HA serum

Peptide serum

Retinol/retinoic acid

Moisturize

Face oil

◆

As a dermatologist I am always interested in the best skincare practices, and I have always had an interest in the anthropological impact on skin care practices that we have records of. The constant evolution of skincare, and the cycling of practices that are founded on basic elements such as oil are fascinating, and potentially beneficial to the readers and patients.

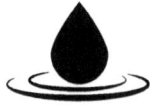

Endnotes

1 https://www.verywellhealth.com/know-your-uv-index-
1069524#:~:text=The%20intensity%20of%20UV%20
radiation%2C%20and%20thus%20the%20UV%20
Index,highest%20in%20spring%20and%20summer

2 https://www.cdc.gov/cancer/skin/
basic_info/sun-safety.htm

3 https://www.skincancer.org/blog/you-missed-a-spot/

4 https://www.skincancer.org/blog/you-missed-a-spot/

5 https://www.ncbi.nlm.nih.gov/
pmc/articles/PMC3583891/

6 https://www.nature.com/articles/d41586-018-07433-7

About the Author

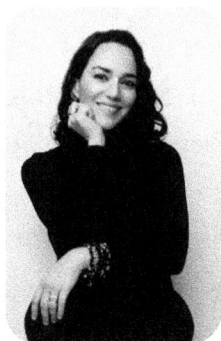

Dr. Kally Papantoniou is a board-certified dermatologist and founder of her proprietary skincare brand Simply Dermatology, and is also a clinical professor at Mount Sinai Hospital in NYC. She is highly specialized in cosmetic dermatology, body contouring, and laser aesthetics, and she practices in New York. She is a featured doctor for *Newbeauty Magazine and has contributed to Glamour, Vogue, Parade, Self, Cosmopolitan & Life & Style magazines.*

As an active member of the American Academy of Dermatology she keeps up with all the latest techniques and cutting-edge approaches to treating her patients. Dr. Papantoniou is meticulous in her work, and in providing her patients with the highest level of care. Delivering skincare with a special interest in natural and healthy alternatives to treatments and disease prevention.

Dr. Papantoniou is a New York trained dermatologist, with an undergraduate degree in Biology and Hellenic studies from New York University and her medical degree from the State University of New York Downstate Medical School. Dr Papantoniou then completed her dermatology residency at State University of New York Downstate Medical Center. She earned her degree in Dermatology with the Award for Excellence in the department.

For more information on Dr. Papantoniou, services offered at Simply Dermatology or her new Simply Oils skin care product visit **www.SimplyDermatology.com**

* 9 7 9 8 9 8 6 2 8 3 0 9 8 *